The Kids' Guide to Disease & Wellness

Why People Get Sick & How They Can Stay Well

CANCER & KIDS

Rae Simons

The Kids' Guide to Disease & Wellness:
Why People Get Sick and How They Can Stay Well
CANCER & KIDS: GET THE FACTS!

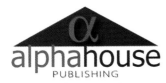

AlphaHouse Publishing
201 Harding Avenue
Vestal, NY 13850

First Printing

9 8 7 6 5 4 3 2 1

ISBN: 978-1-934970-14-0
ISBN (series): 978-1-934970-11-9
   Library of Congress Control Number: 2008930672

Author: Simons, Rae

Cover design by MK Bassett-Harvey.
Interior design by MK Bassett-Harvey and Wendy Arakawa.

Printed in India by International Print-O-Pac Limited

 An ISO 9001 Company

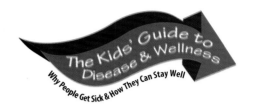

The Kids' Guide to Disease & Wellness
Why People Get Sick & How They Can Stay Well

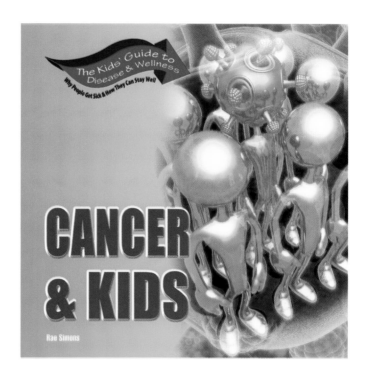

The Kids' Guide to Disease & Wellness
Why People Get Sick & How They Can Stay Well

CANCER & KIDS

Rae Simons

By Rae Simons

Compliments of ...

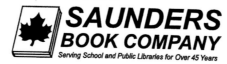

SAUNDERS
BOOK COMPANY
Serving School and Public Libraries for Over 45 Years

Series List

Introduction

According to a recent study reported in the Virginia Henderson International Nursing Library, kids worry about getting sick. They worry about AIDS and cancer, about allergies and the "super-germs" that resist medication. They know about these ills—but they don't always understand what causes them or how they can be prevented.

Unfortunately, most 9- to 11–year–olds, the study found, get their information about diseases like AIDS from friends and television; only 20 percent of the children interviewed based their understanding of illness on facts they had learned at school. Too often, kids believe urban legends, schoolyard folktales, and exaggerated movie plots. Oftentimes, misinformation like this only makes their worries worse. The January 2008 *Child Health News* reported that 55 percent of all children between 9 and 13 "worry almost all the time" about illness.

This series, **The Kids' Guide to Disease and Wellness**, offers readers clear information on various illnesses and conditions, as well as the immunizations that can prevent many diseases. The books dispel the myths with clearly presented facts and colorful, accurate illustrations. Better yet, these books will help kids understand not only illness—but also what they can do to stay as healthy as possible.

—*Dr. Elise Berlan*

Just The Facts

- There are many types of cancer. The one thing they all have in common, however, is that they involve damage to the DNA of cells, which makes these cells grow uncontrollably in the body.

- Cancer cells form things called tumors, which literally squish parts of the body, making people very sick. A tumor starts in one part of the body, but it can spread to other parts.

- Scientists around the world are studying the causes of cancer. Cancer can be caused by pollution, smoking, the sun, and even your genes.

- Doctors have a number of ways to detect cancers, including blood tests, X-rays, and MRIs.

- Cancer is usually treated by cutting out the tumor and then using radiation or chemotherapy treatments.

- There are many people working for a cure for cancer around the world, including famous celebrities.

What Is Cancer?

Cancer is the name for a group of more than 100 diseases. These different diseases all have something in common: cells in a part of the body begin to grow out of control. Untreated cancers can make people very sick and even die.

Normal body cells grow, divide, and die according to schedule. When you're young, your cells divide more quickly, but the process slows down as you become an adult. After that, most of your cells divide only to replace worn-out or dying cells and to repair injuries.

Cancer cells, like the one shown here, start growing when

Words to Know

Environment: All the living and nonliving things that surround us.

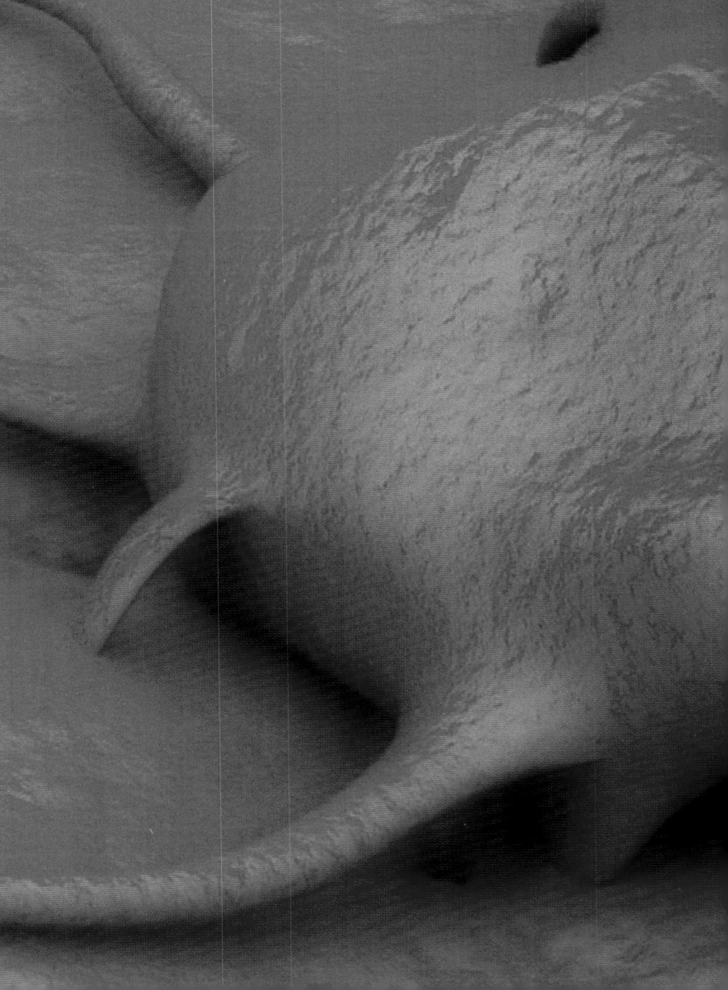

8

the DNA in cells is damaged. DNA is what tells a cell what to do, including when to divide. Usually when DNA is damaged, either the cell dies or it repairs the DNA, but that doesn't happen in cancer cells. People can inherit damaged DNA from their parents, but most often DNA is damaged by things in the environment, like chemicals, viruses, tobacco smoke, or too much sunlight.

ASK THE DOCTOR

My mother has lung cancer. Does that mean I'll get cancer, too?

A: No, it doesn't. Your mother may have cancer because she smoked or because of some other environmental factor that doesn't affect you. If you have two close relatives with cancer, it's possible you too will have a genetic tendency to develop this disease. But even if you have inherited a "cancer gene," that doesn't mean you will definitely get cancer. It just means that if other conditions in the environment are right for cancer, your odds are higher for getting it than other people's are. Living a healthy lifestyle will be even more important.

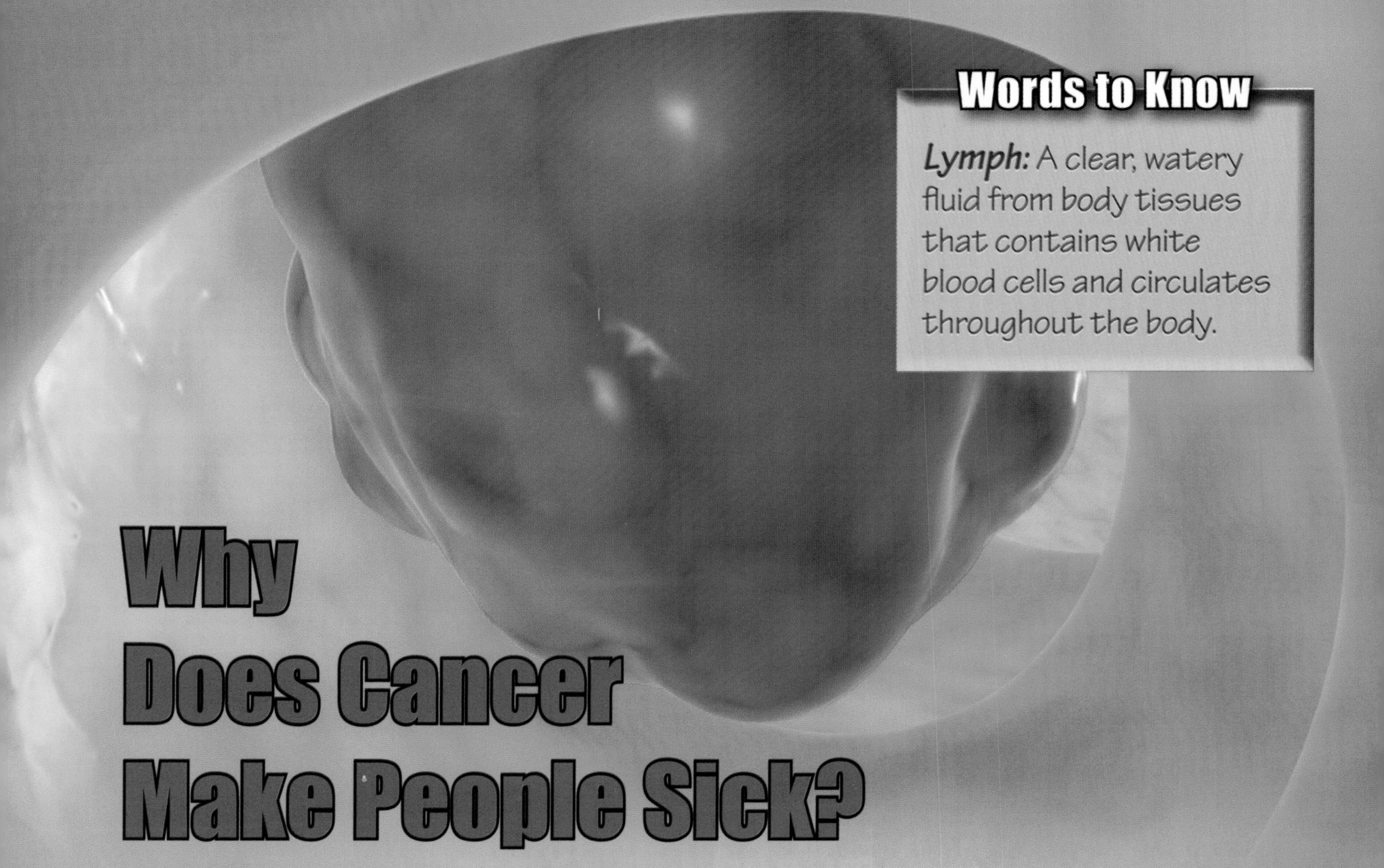

Words to Know

Lymph: A clear, watery fluid from body tissues that contains white blood cells and circulates throughout the body.

Why Does Cancer Make People Sick?

Because cancer cells keep growing and dividing, they outlive normal cells and continue to grow and make new cancer cells. These abnormal cells often form as a tumor (a lump or mass) like the one shown here. These lumps can push on other body organs. The tumors can get in the way. Eventually, organs will be damaged and not be able to do their jobs.

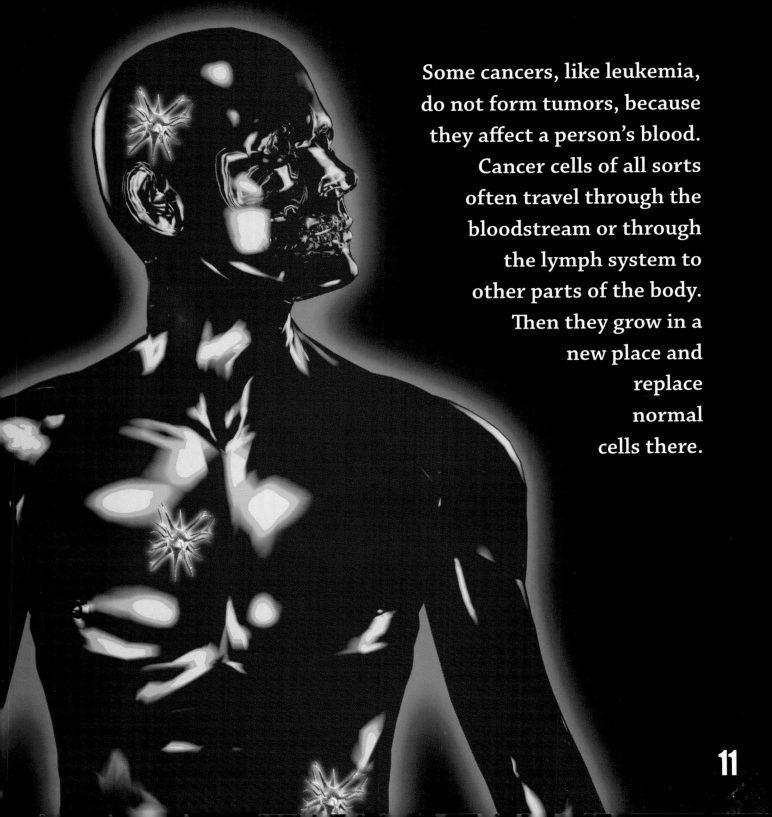

Some cancers, like leukemia, do not form tumors, because they affect a person's blood. Cancer cells of all sorts often travel through the bloodstream or through the lymph system to other parts of the body. Then they grow in a new place and replace normal cells there.

Kinds of Cancer

Cancers that begin in different parts of the body can act very differently from each other. They grow at different rates and respond to different treatments.

Even when cancer has spread to a different part of the body, it is still named for the place in the body where it started. For example, breast cancer that has spread to the liver is metastatic breast cancer, not liver cancer.

Some of the most common kinds of cancer are:

leukemia
lung cancer
skin cancer
colon cancer

Words to Know

Metastatic: having to do with cancer cells spreading through the body.

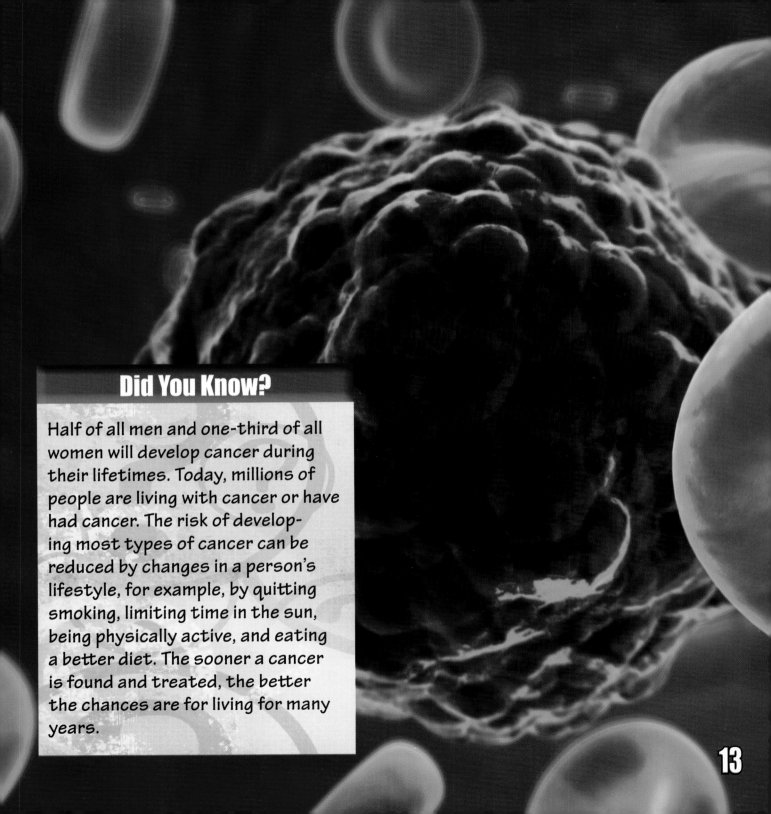

Did You Know?

Half of all men and one-third of all women will develop cancer during their lifetimes. Today, millions of people are living with cancer or have had cancer. The risk of developing most types of cancer can be reduced by changes in a person's lifestyle, for example, by quitting smoking, limiting time in the sun, being physically active, and eating a better diet. The sooner a cancer is found and treated, the better the chances are for living for many years.

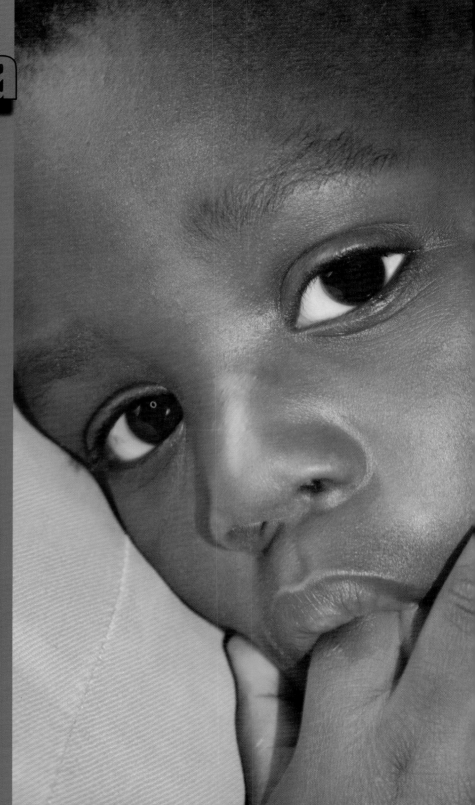

Leukemia

Leukemia is a kind of cancer that affects the white blood cells. It's especially common among children. When someone has leukemia, abnormal white blood cells are produced in the bone marrow. These abnormal white cells crowd the bone marrow and flood the bloodstream, but they cannot do the white blood cells' normal job of protecting the body against disease.

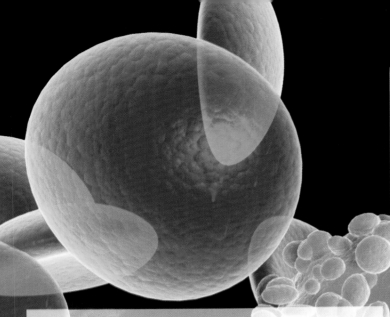
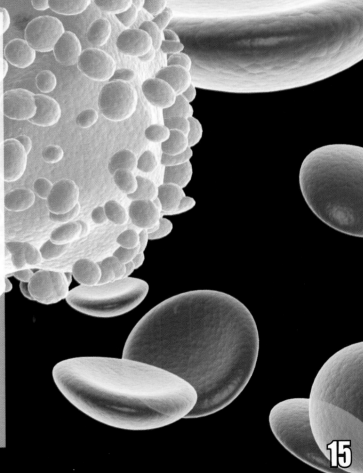

Words to Know

Anemia: a condition where there are fewer healthy red blood cells than normal. Since red blood cells carry the oxygen your body's cells need for energy, anemia can make you feel tired and weak.

As leukemia progresses, it interferes with the body's production of other types of blood cells, including red blood cells. This results in anemia and bleeding problems, as well as an increased risk of catching other infections.

Luckily, the chances for a cure are very good with leukemia. With treatment, most children with leukemia are free of the disease without it coming back.

Lung Cancer

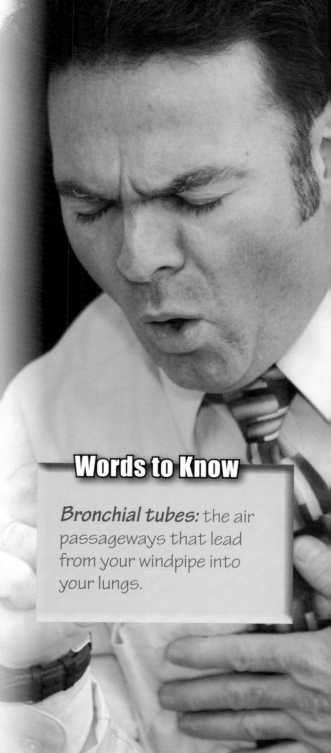

Lung cancer is caused by abnormal cells growing in the lungs, usually in the cells lining the air passageways, including the bronchial tubes. This growth may eventually invade the body parts around the lungs as well. It can also metastasize and spread through the body.

Lung cancer is the most common cause of cancer-related death in men and the second most common in women. Around the world, 1.3 million people die from it each year.

The most common symptoms of lung cancer are shortness of breath, coughing (including coughing up blood), and weight loss.

Words to Know

Bronchial tubes: the air passageways that lead from your windpipe into your lungs.

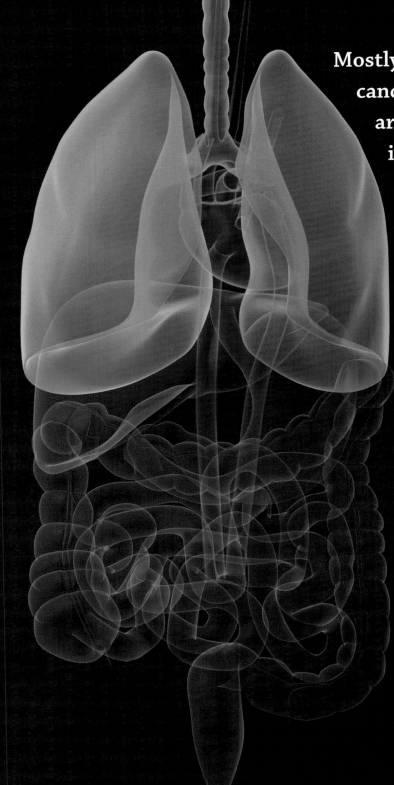

Mostly older people get lung cancer—and 90 percent of them are smokers. (In other words, if you have a group of 10 people with lung cancer, 9 of them would probably smoke.) Before the 1930s, lung cancer was very rare, but as cigarettes became popular around the world, the numbers of people with lung cancer shot up. Among those who smoke two or more packs of cigarettes per day, one in seven will die of lung cancer.

Today, people in many countries are being educated about the risks of smoking, and the cases of lung cancer are becoming fewer.

Skin Cancer

Skin cancer is the abnormal growth of skin cells. It most often develops on skin exposed to the sun, but sometimes it can also occur on areas of your skin not ordinarily in the sun.

Most skin cancers can be prevented if you protect your skin from the sun's harmful rays. You should also pay attention to any changes to your skin, including any new spots (or spots that have changed in color or shape). Skin cancer can be treated successfully if you catch it early.

Words to Know

Exposed: placed where a condition or action can affect or change something.

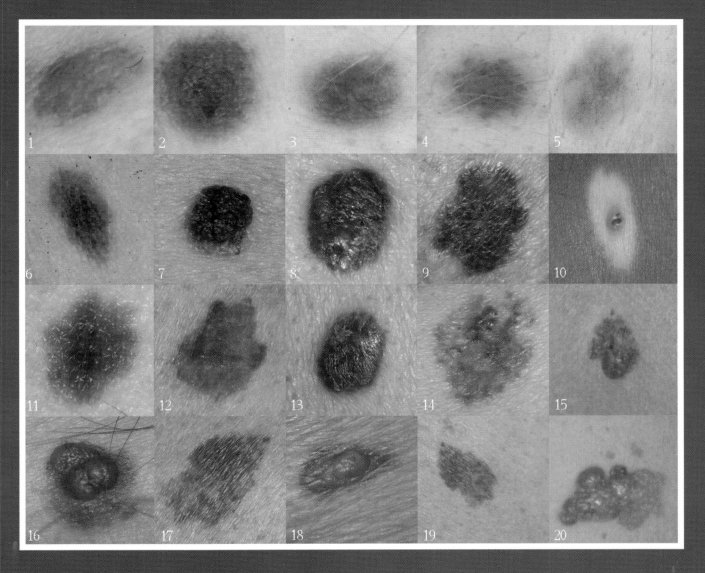

These are all examples of moles that are actually skin cancer. Tell a grownup (and go see your doctor) if you have a mole that gets bigger, changes shape, or changes color. Not all spots on your skin are cancer—but only a doctor can tell you for sure.

Colon Cancer

Words to Know

Polyp: a mass of tissue that develops on the inside of a hollow body organ.

A person with colon cancer will have cancerous tumors in the colon (like the one shown to the right). Your colon is the tube through which waste materials pass from your stomach and small intestine and eventually into the toilet. Your colon is also sometimes called your large intestine.

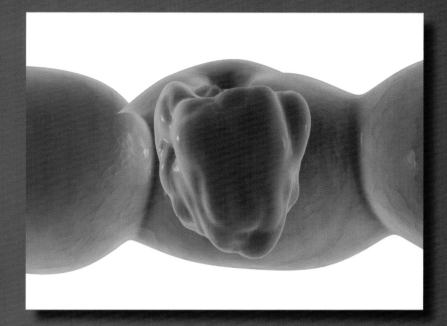

Most colon cancers start out as harmless polyps like the one shown to the left. These slowly change into cancer, but scientists are not sure why. Diet may play a role. Scientists believe that eating plenty of whole grains and other high-fiber foods may help keep your colon healthy.

See a doctor if you notice any change in your bowel movement habits.

Did You Know?

Colon cancer is the third most common form of cancer and the second leading cause of cancer-related death in Europe and North America. Colon cancer causes 655,000 deaths worldwide each year.

cancer and Genes

Scientists around the world are working hard to understand what causes cancer. They want to understand how a normal cell can turn into a cancerous cell through a series of changes in its genes. Scientists have found that certain genes play a part in some cancers. When people are born with a gene change (mutation) that makes them more likely to develop cancer, scientists say they have inherited a cancer gene.

This mutation may then also be passed on to their children.

There are two types of genetic changes or mutations: those that are passed down from generation to generation, and those that happen during the lifetime of a person and are not passed on to the next generation. Inherited genes become a part of you at the moment of conception. Because all the cells of your body develop from one fertilized egg, all the cells in your body will contain the genetic change that puts you at risk of getting cancer.

Words to Know

Gene: the unit of inheritance contained on a chromosome (the spiral shape shown on the page to the left), which contains the directions for new cell formation.

Conception: the moment when an egg is fertilized with a sperm with the potential to become a new person or animal.

Cancer and the Environment

The good news is that most cancers are not inherited. As many as two-thirds of all cancer cases are linked to environmental causes. This means if we can change the environment, we can prevent these cancers.

Did You Know?

Scientists have found that people who live in the world's most polluted cities are much more likely to die at a younger age than those in cities with the cleanest air.

Cancer clusters are places where many people have cancer, usually because of an environmental factor.

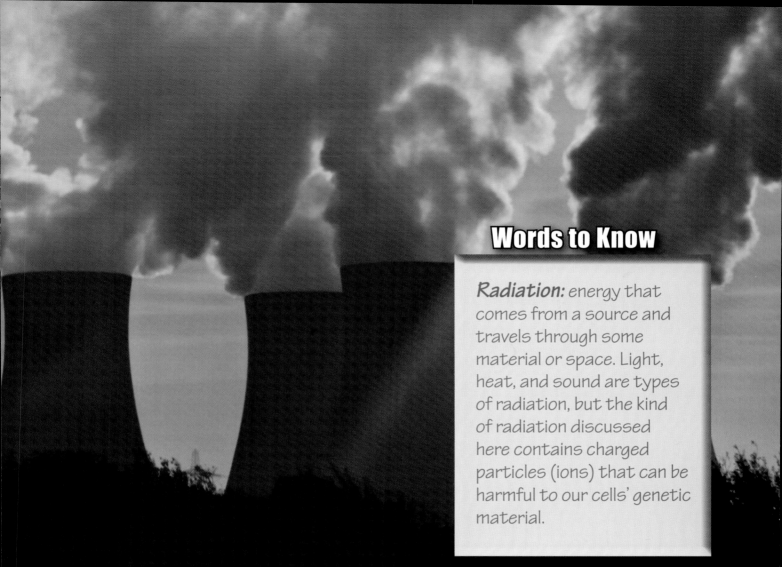

Words to Know

Radiation: energy that comes from a source and travels through some material or space. Light, heat, and sound are types of radiation, but the kind of radiation discussed here contains charged particles (ions) that can be harmful to our cells' genetic material.

Pollution increases our risk of getting cancer. Factories, cars, farms, and buildings release chemicals and radiation into our air, water, food, and homes. When we take these chemicals into our bodies through our lungs, our mouths, and our skin, we expose our bodies' cells to substances that can trigger the genetic cell changes that cause cancer.

Cancer and Lifestyle
dangerous sunshine

Most of us love sunshine. The sun's rays make us feel good. But sunshine isn't always good for us. In fact, it can cause cancer. The sun's ultraviolet (UV) radiation is the number-one cause of skin cancer. It triggers changes in skin cells' genes which can eventually turn into cancer. And it doesn't matter how hot it is—being out in the sun too much during the winter puts you at the same risk as being in the sun in the summer.

The more times you've had a severe sunburn before you're 18, the more likely you are to have a serous form of skin cancer when you're older. Being out in the sun day after day, year after year, may give you a nice tan—but it also can cause a less serious form of skin cancer.

ASK THE DOCTOR

My friends say that a safer way to get a suntan is to go to a tanning salon, where you won't even have to be in the sun to get a nice tan. Are they right?

A: No, they're not! Tanning beds also use ultraviolet rays to give you a tan—which means they can also cause skin cancer.

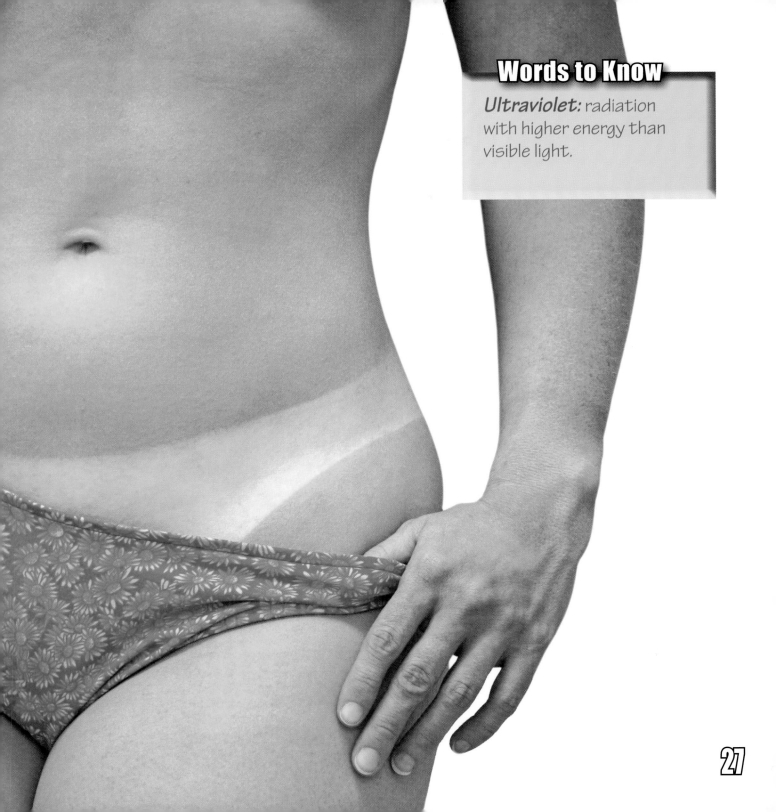

Words to Know

Ultraviolet: radiation with higher energy than visible light.

27

Cancer and Lifestyle

Smoking

Did You Know?

Tobacco use causes more than 5 million deaths worldwide each year. If people keep smoking this much, tobacco use will cause more than 8 million deaths a year by 2030. On average, smokers die 13 to 14 years earlier than non-smokers.

The chemicals found in tobacco smoke also trigger changes in body cells that can lead to cancer. In fact, smoking damages nearly every organ in the human body. Scientists have linked smoking to at least 15 different cancers. At least 30 percent of all deaths caused by cancer (that's about one-third) are caused by smoking. When it comes to lung cancer, the numbers are even worse: smoking causes 90 percent of all lung cancers.

So if you don't want to get lung cancer, there's something doctors know will help: don't smoke! And if you do smoke, quit! Smoking is the world's most preventable cause of death.

ASK THE DOCTOR

My dad smokes all the time. How dangerous is it that I breathe his smoke?

A: It's pretty dangerous. You need to ask your father not to smoke around you—and if he won't listen to you, whenever you can, open the window and leave the house until it's aired out. Let your father know that scientists have discovered that people who live with secondhand smoke all the time are very likely to develop lung cancer and other smoking-related cancers.

Words to Know

Organ: a part of the body that carries out one or more special functions (such as your heart or lungs).

Diagnosing Cancer Symptoms

Even thinking about cancer can make people feel scared. So some people don't like to think about cancer's warning signs. They'd rather just not think about anything to do with cancer until they have to!

But since so many cancers respond well to early treatment, finding out as soon as possible if you have cancer is very important. The sooner you know, the sooner you can begin treatment.

So keep an eye open for the seven symptoms listed on the next page. It's not a scary thing. It's a way to stay safe!

Words to Know

Discharge: flow of fluid from a part of the body.

The 7 Warning ! Signs of Cancer

1. Unusual bleeding or discharge from any part of your body.

2. A sore that doesn't heal.

3. A change in your bathroom habits.

4. A lump in your flesh.

5. A cough that doesn't go away.

6. A change in the shape or color of a mole.

7. Difficulty swallowing.

If you have any of these symptoms, tell a grownup—and make sure you see a doctor right away.

ASK THE DOCTOR

We just found out that my grandmother has breast cancer. Does that mean she's going to die?

A: No, it doesn't. Most women who get treatment for their cancer will live at least another five years. Many women will recover completely. It all depends on what kind of cancer your grandmother has and how soon it was found. Her doctor will be able to answer your questions so you know better what to expect.

Blood Tests

Blood tests alone usually can't tell a doctor if you have cancer. But they can give your doctor clues about what's going on inside your body. A nurse or technician will take a little blood from your arm

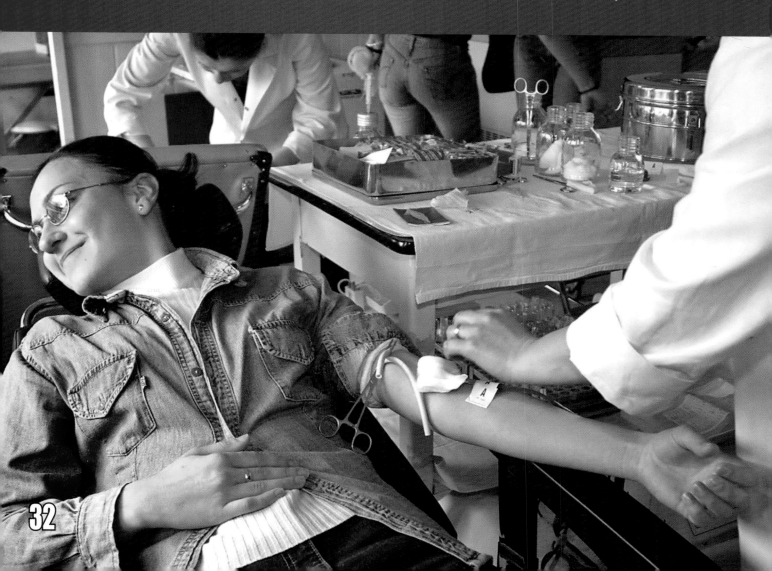

and then do various tests on it in a lab. If the doctor finds cancer cells, too many or too few cells of a certain type, or abnormal types of cells, she may want you to have more tests.

For most forms of cancer, a biopsy—a procedure that cuts out a few suspicious cells for testing—is usually necessary before the doctor can know for sure. Sometimes the doctor will order other tests that allow her to "look inside" your body and see if anything is there that shouldn't be.

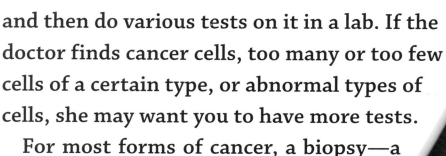

Words to Know

Lab: laboratory, a place with the equipment needed for scientific research.

Procedure: a course of action undertaken to achieve a particular result.

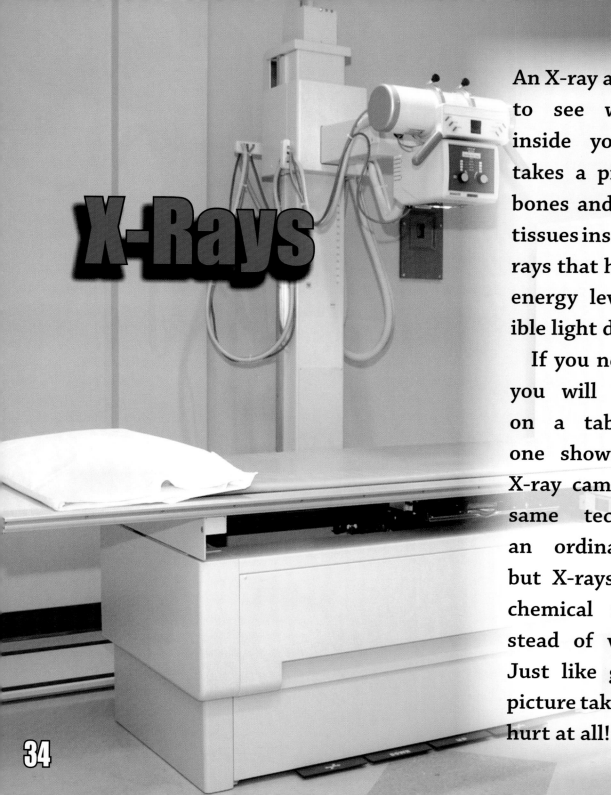

X-Rays

An X-ray allows doctors to see what's going inside your body. It takes a picture of the bones and some of the tissues inside you, using rays that have a higher energy level than visible light does.

If you need an X-ray, you will probably lie on a table like the one shown here. The X-ray camera uses the same technology as an ordinary camera, but X-rays set off the chemical reaction instead of visible light. Just like getting your picture taken, it doesn't hurt at all!

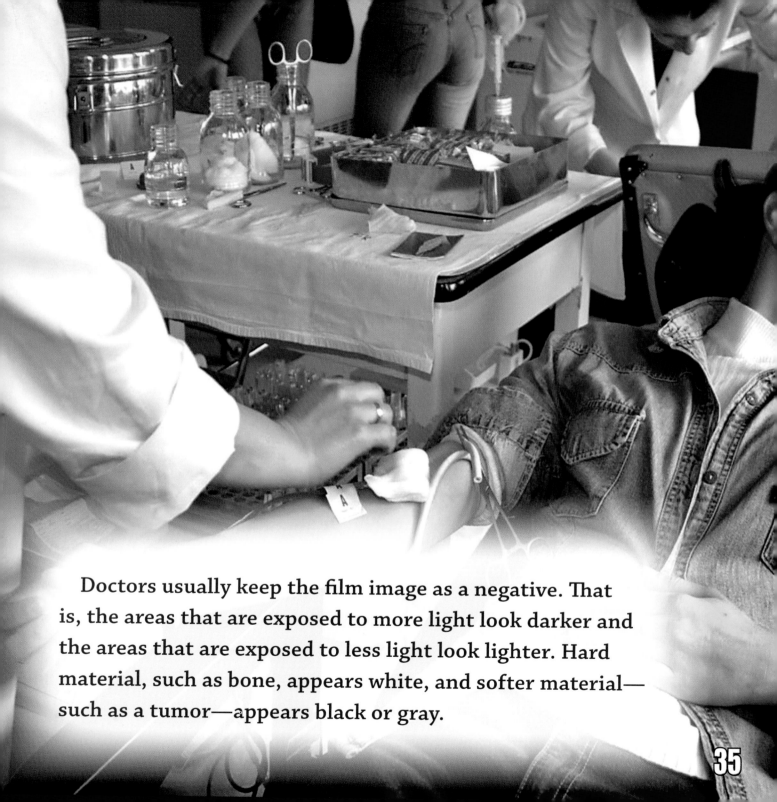

Doctors usually keep the film image as a negative. That is, the areas that are exposed to more light look darker and the areas that are exposed to less light look lighter. Hard material, such as bone, appears white, and softer material—such as a tumor—appears black or gray.

CAT Scans and MRIs

CAT scans use a special type of X-ray. The patient lies down on a couch that slides into a large circle-shaped opening. The X-ray tube rotates around the patient and a computer collects the results. These results are turned into images that look like a "slice" of the person.

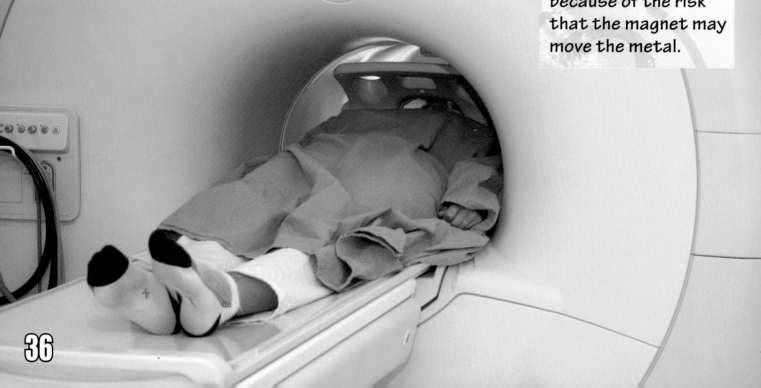

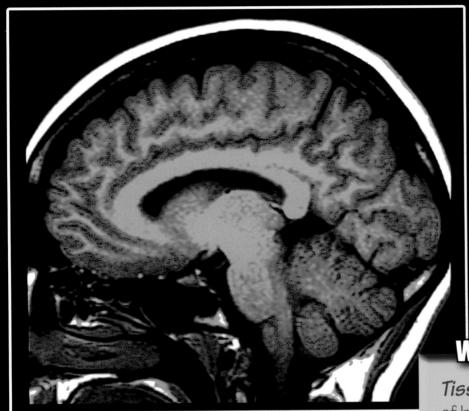

If you have an MRI, you will go inside a very long cylinder. You will be asked to stay perfectly still for about 30 minutes while the machine makes a lot of noise .

The cylinder you lie in is actually a very large magnet. Radio waves are sent through your body and a computer collects the signals and turns them into images. These images look similar to a CAT scan but they have much higher detail in the soft tissues. This means they are useful for discovering tumors and other abnormal masses. But the only way to know for sure if a tumor is cancer is to cut out a little piece during surgery and test it.

Cancer Treatment

If you find out that you or someone you love has cancer, it's normal to feel scared and sad. But scientists and doctors have found many ways to treat cancer.

Getting cancer doesn't have to mean you're going to die! It probably will mean, though, that you spend some time in a hospital. You may not have to sleep there, but you will probably have to visit often to receive the treatments you need.

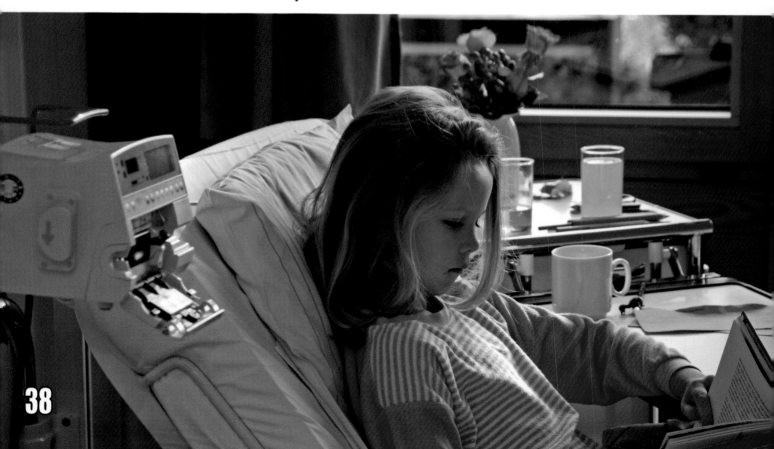

If you have cancer, your body's immune system will be working hard to destroy the invaders in your body—the cancer cells that don't belong there. Cancer treatments help your body do its job better.

There are three main kinds of cancer treatment:

- surgery
- radiation treatment
- chemotherapy

Your doctor will help you decide which is best.

Words to Know

Immune system: the group of body parts that defends your body against diseases and infections.

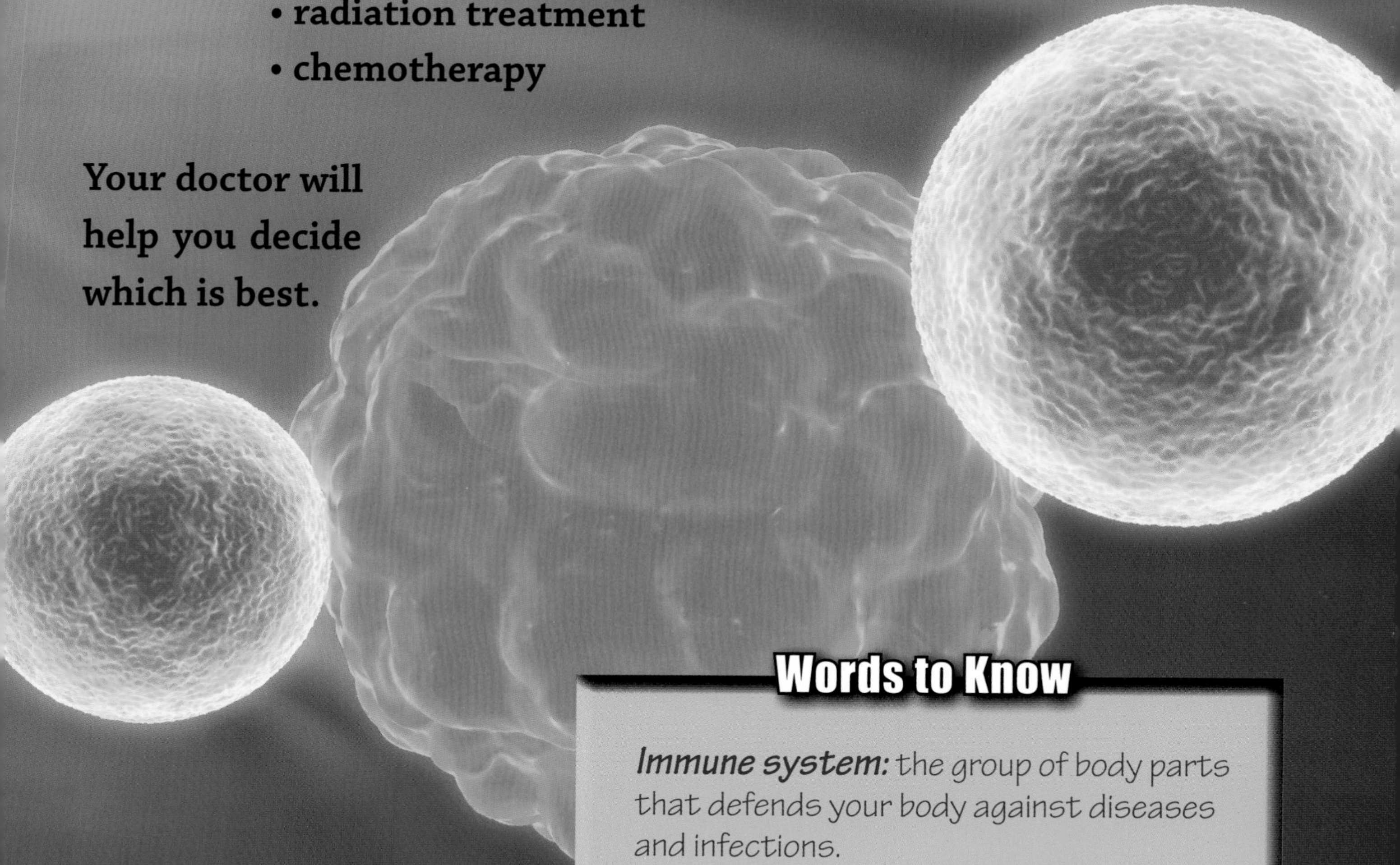

Oncologists

Oncologists are special cancer doctors, and oncology is the branch of medicine that studies tumors (cancer). Oncologists try to understand cancer's development, diagnosis, treatment, and prevention. Oncologists often coordinate the complete care of cancer patients. This may involve physiotherapy, counseling, and genetic counseling.

Did You Know?

The word "oncology" comes from a Greek word— "onkos"— that means mass or tumor. The end of the word— "ology"—is from another Greek word that means "study of."

Oncologists are also the doctors who diagnose whether someone has cancer. They're the doctors who oversee cancer treatment. After treatment is over, they also follow up with cancer patients, checking them regularly to make sure they stay healthy.

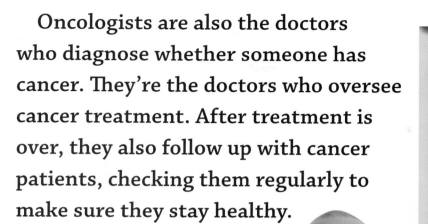
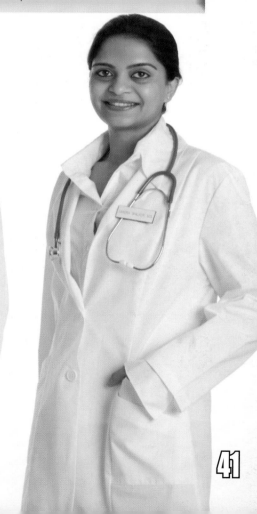

41

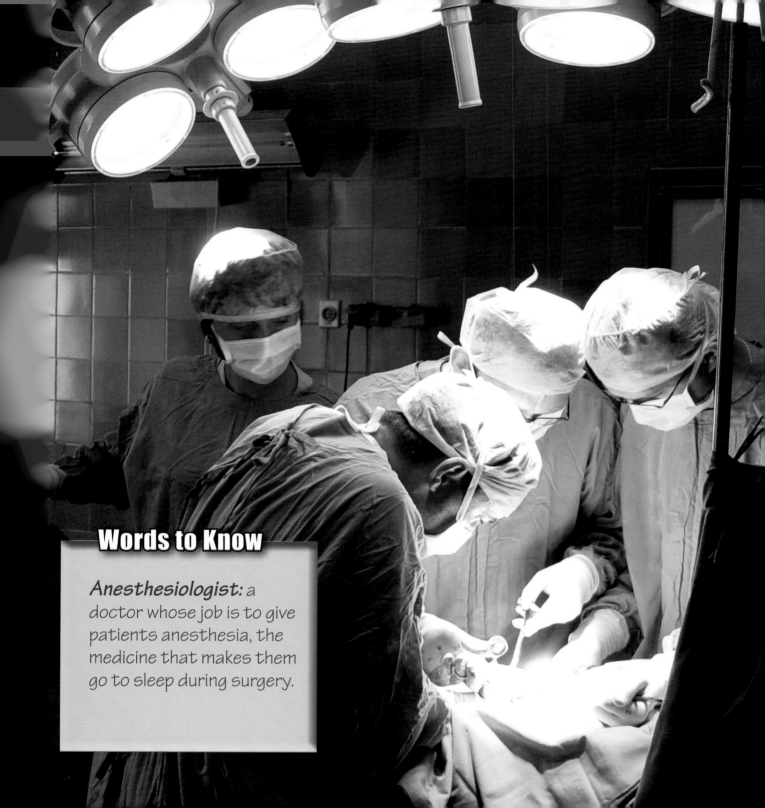

Words to Know

Anesthesiologist: a doctor whose job is to give patients anesthesia, the medicine that makes them go to sleep during surgery.

Surgery

Surgery is the oldest form of cancer treatment. It is also an important part of diagnosing cancer and finding out how far it has spread.

If you need to have a surgery, you will probably be admitted into a hospital. One of the workers in the hospital will take you to the operating room. Oftentimes you will go there on a special bed with wheels. The room will have bright lights on the ceiling, and while you are there, a special doctor called an anesthesiologist willl give you medicine that makes you go to sleep. When you wake up, the surgery will be over.

Surgery is the best way to cure many types of cancer, especially those that have not spread to other parts of the body.

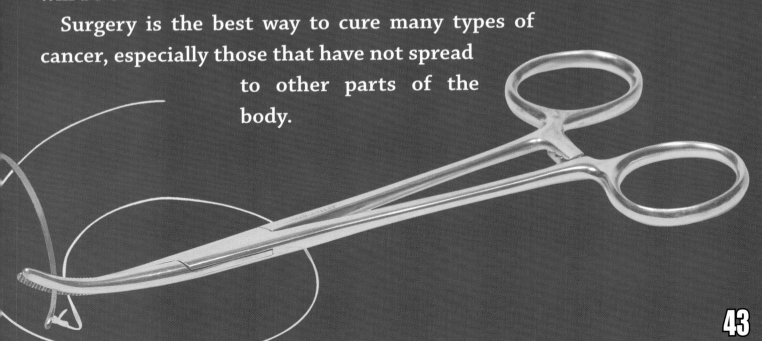

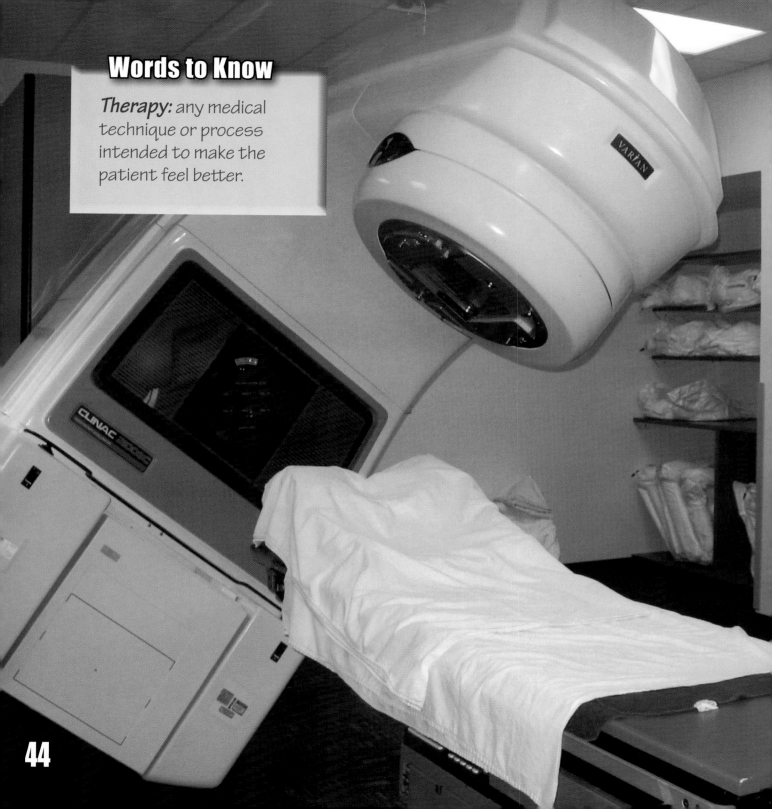

Words to Know

Therapy: any medical technique or process intended to make the patient feel better.

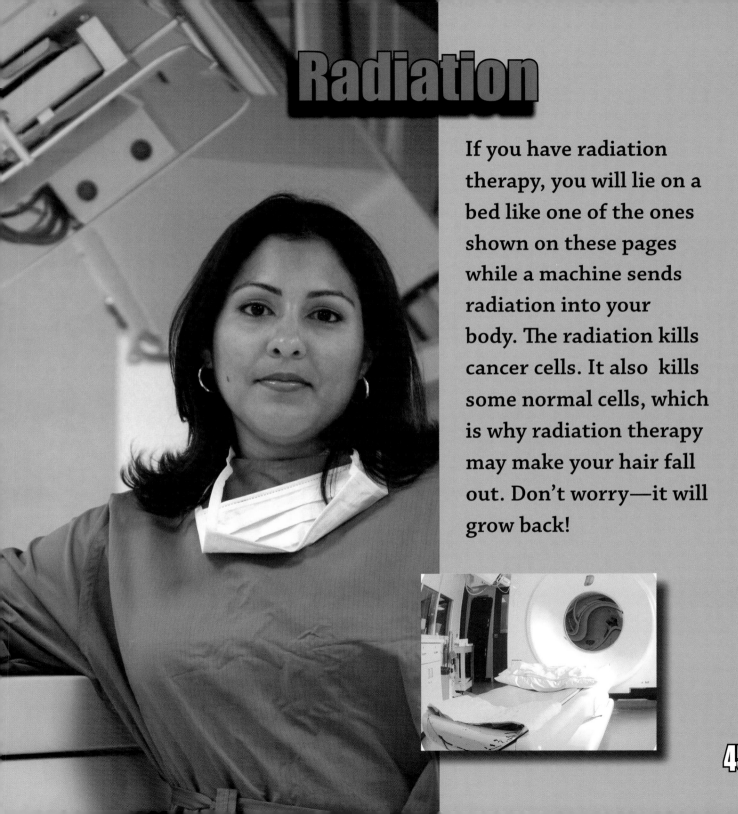

Radiation

If you have radiation therapy, you will lie on a bed like one of the ones shown on these pages while a machine sends radiation into your body. The radiation kills cancer cells. It also kills some normal cells, which is why radiation therapy may make your hair fall out. Don't worry—it will grow back!

45

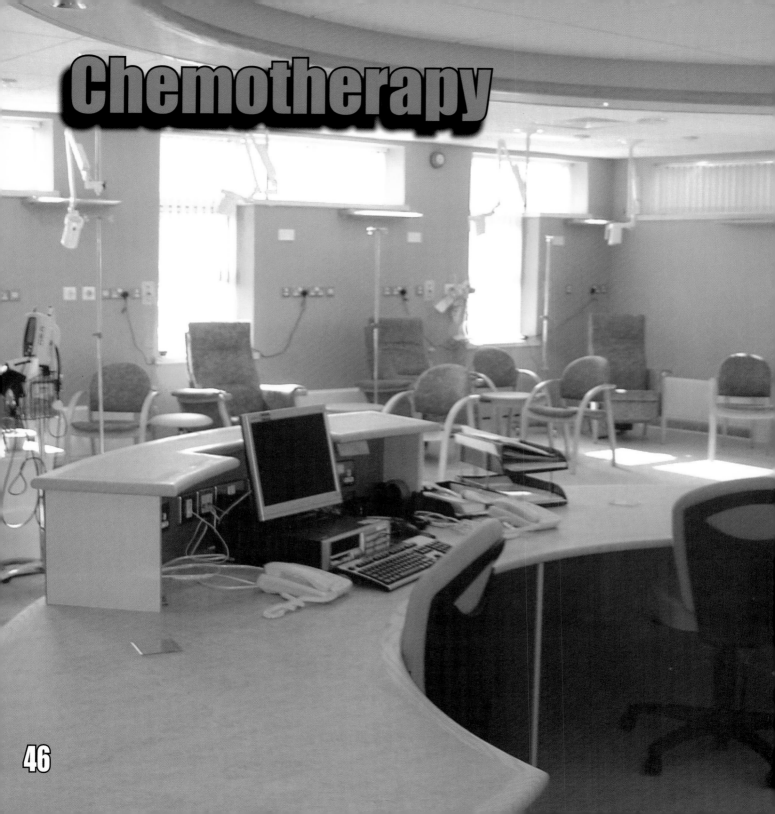

Chemotherapy

Chemotherapy— "chemo" for short—most often means taking certain types of medicines to treat cancer. You might take these drugs before or after cancer surgery. You might take them along with radiation treatment. Or you might take the medicines alone. Your oncologist will decide what is the best treatment for the kind of cancer you have.

During chemotherapy, you may go into a hospital every week or every few weeks. While the medicine is being given to you (often through a tube that carries it into one of your blood vessels), you will sit in a chair, probably in a room that looks a little like the one on the page to the left.

Because the chemicals in the medicine affect both cancer cells and normal cells, chemotherapy often makes people feel sick. It is an important weapon in the battle against cancer, though. Because of it, many people with cancer will have full, healthy lives when their treatment is completed.

Did You Know?

While surgery and radiation therapy attack cancer cells directly in a specific area, chemotherapy works throughout the entire body. Its goal is to destroy cancer cells wherever they may be, even if they have spread to parts of the body far from the original tumor. Chemotherapy destroys cancer cells by interfering with their growth, by preventing them from reproducing, and, in some cases, by reprogramming the cells so they make themselves die.

Bone Marrow Transplants

When people have certain kinds of cancer, especially leukemia, cancer attacks their bone marrow. This can make them very sick. A bone marrow transplant takes bone marrow from a healthy person and puts it into a patient whose bone marrow is not working properly. This is one way to treat leukemia and other cancers.

Donated bone marrow must match the patient's tissue type. It is often taken from a close relative.

Bone marrow is taken from the donor in an operating room while the donor is asleep from anesthesia. Some of the donor's bone marrow is removed from the top of the hip bone. Then it will be put into the other person.

Alternative Treatments

Many people with cancer want to try treatments besides the ones we've mentioned here. These are sometimes called "alternative treatments." They include things like herbal medicines, meditation techniques, and traditional Asian medicines. Not all these treatments are safe, however, and most of them have very little effect on cancer. Doctors suggest that cancer patients use alternative cancer treatments as a supplement to treatments they receive from their doctors—not as a substitute for medical care.

Alternative cancer treatments can help patients cope with pain and discomfort, but they generally aren't strong enough to replace medications from a doctor. The following techniques may be helpful, though:

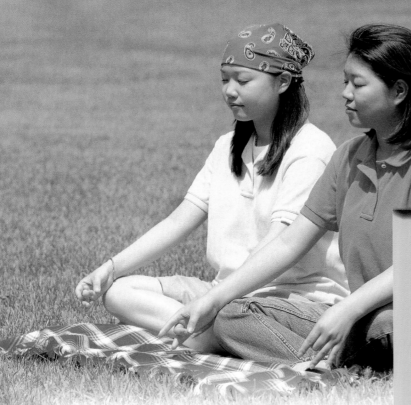

Words to Know

Supplement: something added to complete the whole.

Yoga: a system of exercises to promote control of the body and mind that are based on a Hindu religious practice.

Acupuncture: a procedure from Chinese medical practice in which specific body areas are pierced with fine needles to relieve pain.

- Yoga can help sleep problems and improve energy levels during cancer treatment.
- Acupuncture can help reduce nausea from chemotherapy and diminish pain.
- Meditation and prayer can help cancer patients cope with anxiety, stress, and depression.

Research

Did You Know?

In April 2008, the Russian Ministry of Public Health approved the world's first kidney cancer vaccine. The vaccine will help prevent kidney cancer from coming back once a patient has been successfully treated.

Scientists around the world are working to find better ways to prevent, treat, and cure cancer. They work in labs and look through microscopes, they do experiments on animals and cells, and they carefully watch how people respond to different treatments. Their work is helping them better understand what causes cancer—and what can be done to both cure it and prevent it from happening. The more scientists understand about cancer, the more weapons doctors will have to fight it.

Words to Know

Vaccine: a substance that causes the immune system to be able to better fight off invaders, such as cancer cells or germs like bacteria and viruses. A vaccine is often given as a "shot."

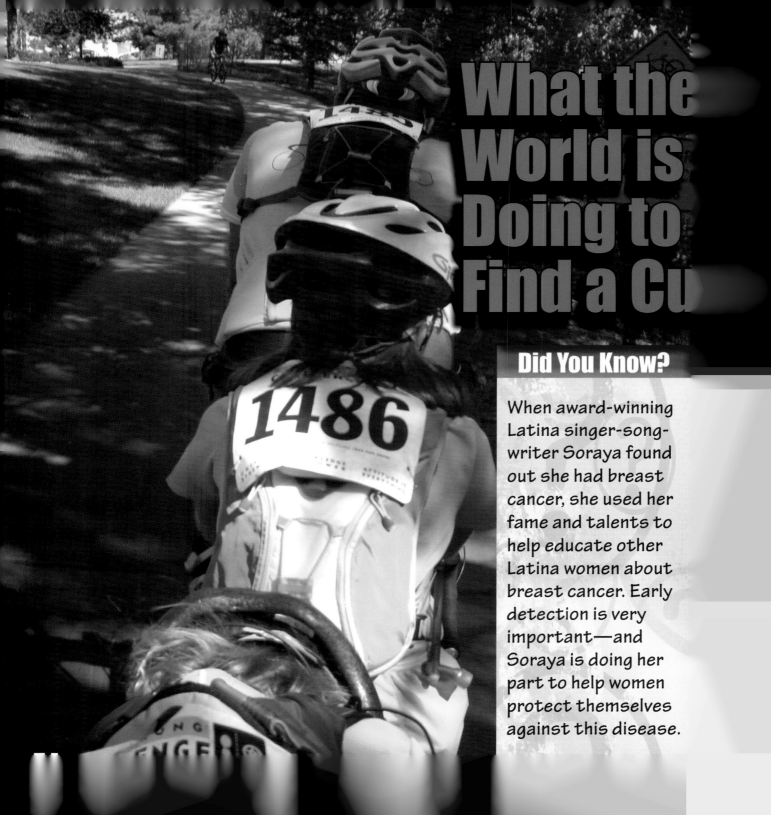

What the World is Doing to Find a Cu

Did You Know?

When award-winning Latina singer-song-writer Soraya found out she had breast cancer, she used her fame and talents to help educate other Latina women about breast cancer. Early detection is very important—and Soraya is doing her part to help women protect themselves against this disease.

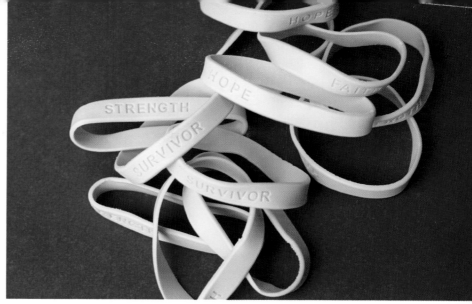

Cancer affects everyone. Almost everyone in the world knows someone who has had this disease. That is why people around the world are becoming activists in the fight against cancer. Organizations like Livestrong, founded by cyclist Lance Armstrong who won his own battle against cancer, get people involved in raising money for cancer research and promoting awareness. They do this by organizing marathons and bike rides. Bracelets like the ones shown on this page also draw attention to breast cancer and other cancer causes. According to the Livestrong Web site, when it comes to fighting cancer, unity is strength, knowledge is power, and attitude is everything!

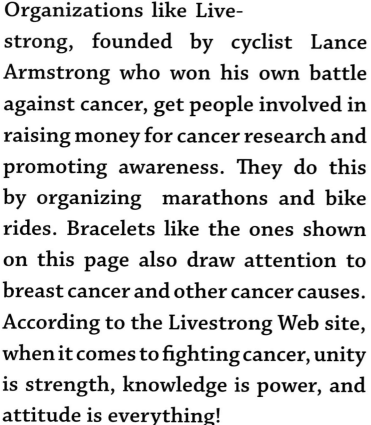

Words to Know

Detection: finding out about something.

Activists: people who take action to bring about some change in the world.

Marathons: long-distance races.

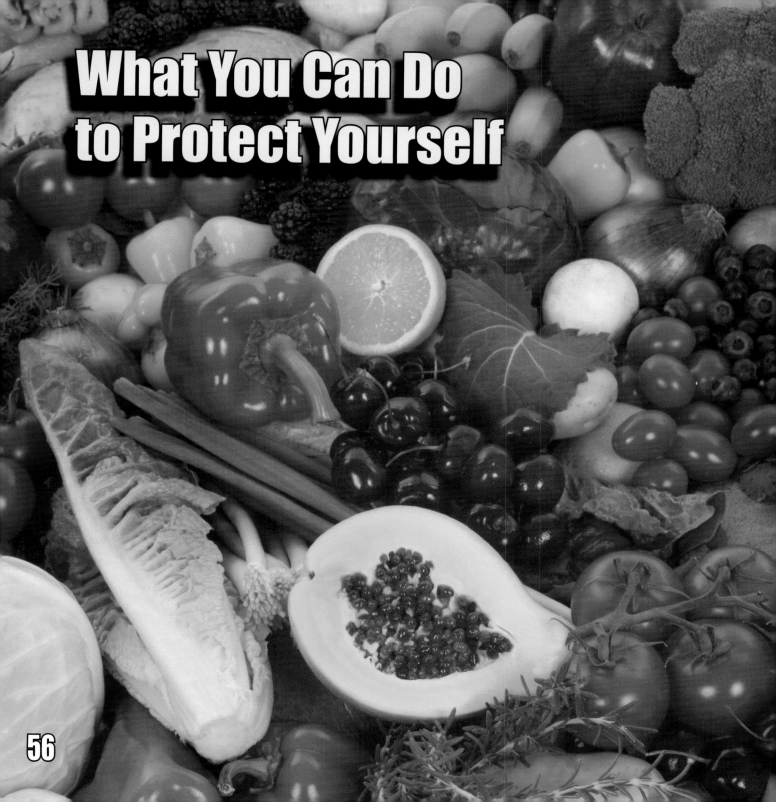

What You Can Do to Protect Yourself

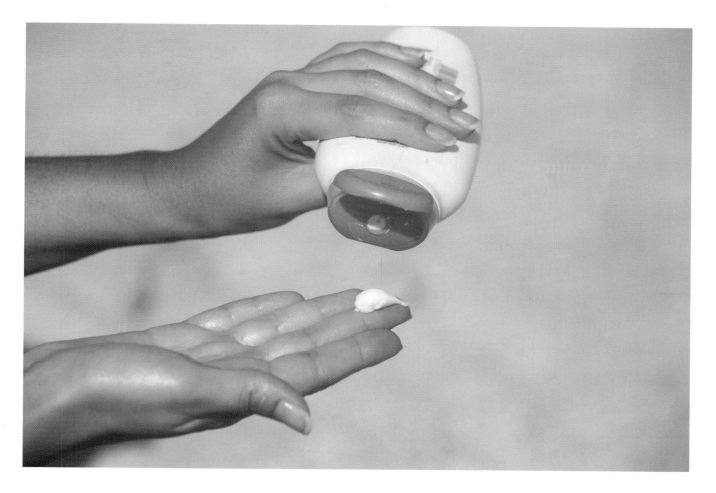

Cancer is a scary disease—but you can take steps to protect yourself against it. One of the best ways to prevent cancer is to eat a healthy diet that includes plenty of fruits and vegetables. These foods contain chemicals that can actually help your body fight off the dangerous substances that can trigger cancer in your body's cells. You can also protect yourself by using sunscreen when you're out in the sun. And one of the best ways of all? Don't smoke!

Real Kids

Jamie Stafford's mom found out her son had leukemia when he was only 8 months old. The entire family's life changed after that. Jamie had to be in the hospital for weeks at a time for treatment. Sometimes Jamie's treatments made him sick, too. He would just come home, only to have a bad reaction to a medicine he was taking and have to go back in the hospital.

Jamie's older sister Amanda also had a tough time through all this. She was worried about her baby brother, and it made her sad to see him in the hospital. But she also felt lonely

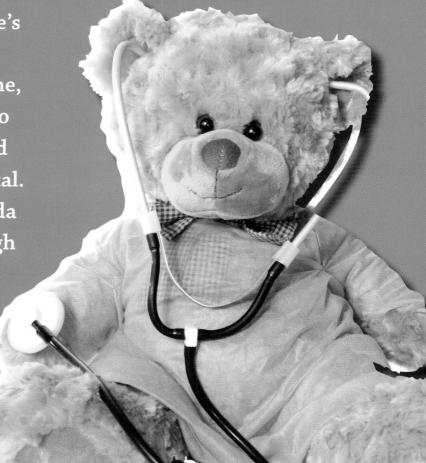

sometimes because her mother needed to spend so much time with Jamie. There wasn't much time left over for Amanda. Sometimes Amanda felt angry and jealous—and then she felt guilty. Amanda's feelings were perfectly normal, though, and she had nothing to feel guilty about.

Today, after three long years of treatment, Jamie is finally healthy again. Amanda's glad to have her baby brother back home for good.

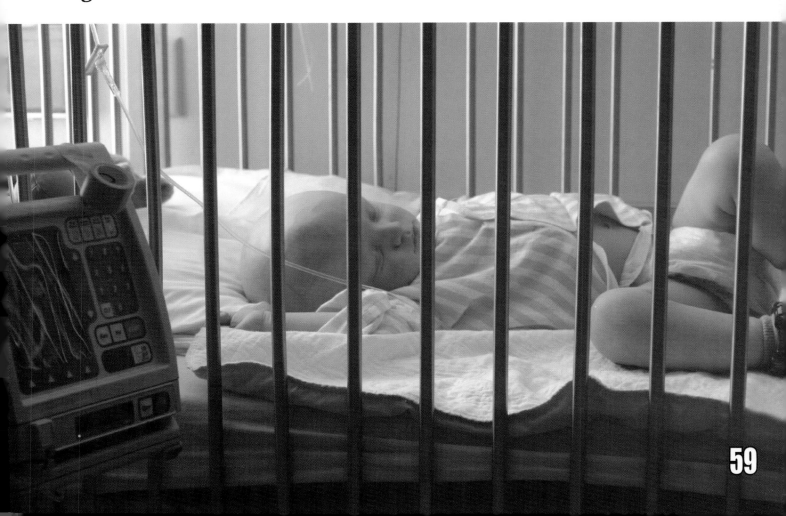

Find Out More

American Cancer Society

www.cancer.org

Cancer Kids

www.cancerkids.org

Cancer Information

www.oncolink.com

Cancer Research UK

info.cancerresearchuk.org

Childhood Cancer

www.kidshealth.org/parent/medical/cancer/cancer.html

Children's Cancer Web

www.cancerindex.org/ccw/guide2y.htm

Mayo Clinic Cancer Awareness
www.mayoclinic.com/health/cancer/CA00055

National Cancer Institute
www.cancer.gov

World Health Organization/Cancer
www.who.int/cancer

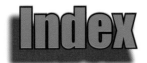

Index

Picture Credits

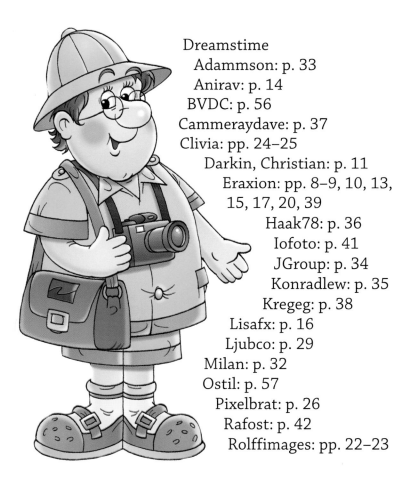

About the Author

Rae Simons has written many books for young adults and children. She lives in upstate New York with her family.

About the Consultant

Elise DeVore Berlan, MD, MPH, FAAP, is a faculty member of the Division of Adolescent Health at Nationwide Children's Hospital and an Assistant Professor of Clinical Pediatrics at The Ohio State University College of Medicine. She completed her Fellowship in Adolescent Medicine at Children's Hospital Boston and obtained a Master's Degree in Public Health at the Harvard School of Public Health. Dr. Berlan completed her residency in pediatrics at the Children's Hospital of Philadelphia, where she also served an additional year as Chief Resident. She received her medical degree from the University of Iowa College of Medicine. Dr. Berlan is board certified in Pediatrics and board eligible in Adolescent Medicine. She provides primary care and consultative services in the area of Young Women's Health, including gynecological problems, concerns about puberty, reproductive health services, and reproductive endocrine disorders.